ANEMIA DIET COOKBOOK

Overcoming Anemia: 50+ Delicious and Nutrient-Packed Recipes for a Sustainable, Healthy Life – Your Essential Guide to Boosting Iron Levels

Rosalie M. Johnson

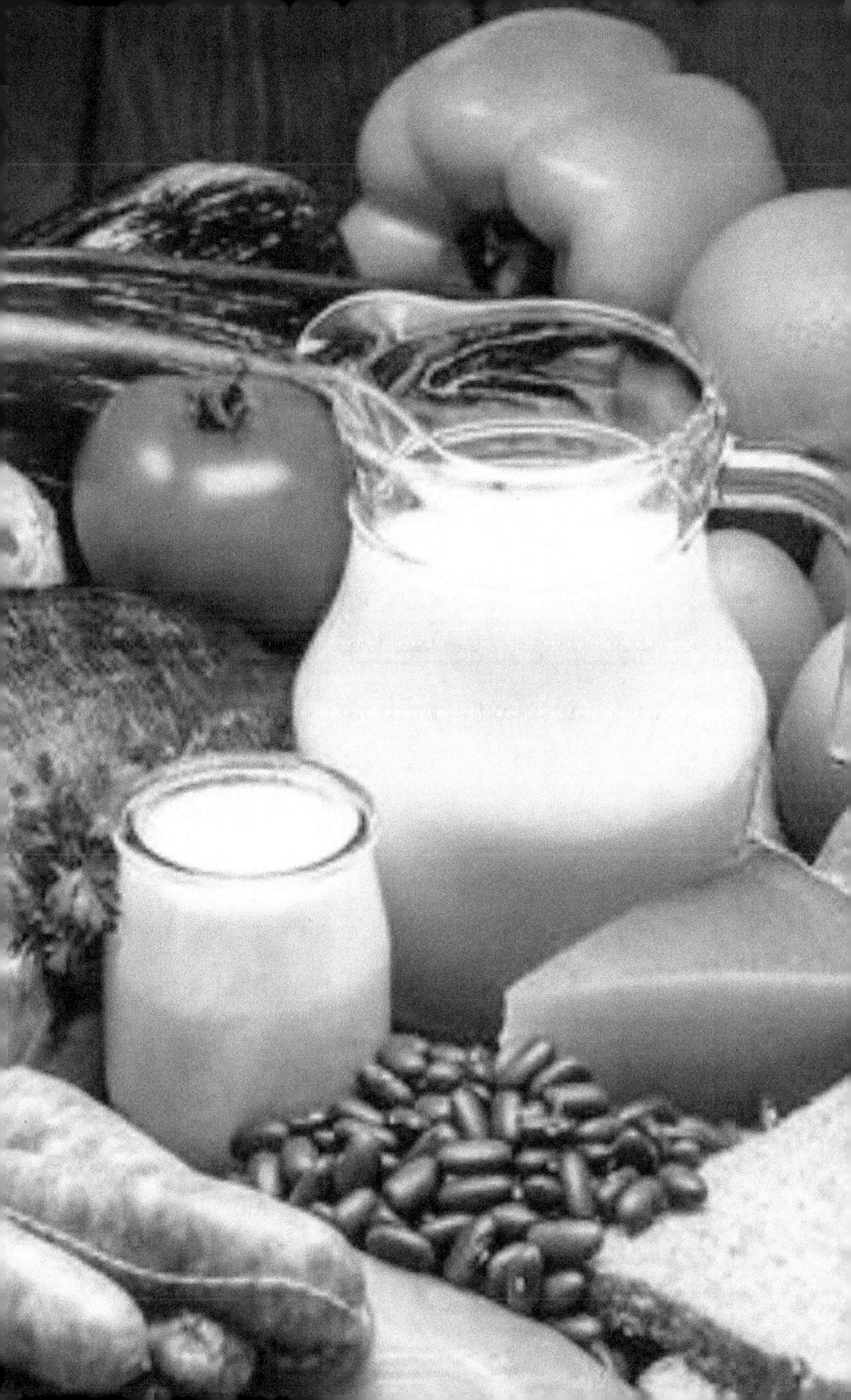

INTRODUCTION

Understanding Anemia

Once upon a time, in a bustling kitchen filled with the aroma of freshly chopped herbs and sizzling pans, there lived a curious cook. She wasn't just any cook; she was on a mission—a mission to understand the silent villain that plagued millions worldwide: anemia.

The Whispering Fatigue

She had always been passionate about food. She reveled in the alchemy of flavors, the dance of spices, and the art of nourishing others. But lately, something was amiss. Her once boundless energy had dwindled to a mere flicker. The vibrant hues of her culinary creations seemed muted, and her zest for life waned like a fading sunset.

"Why?" she wondered, stirring a pot of lentil soup. "Why does fatigue cling to me like a shadow? Why do my steps feel heavier, as if I carry the weight of a thousand cast-iron skillets?"

The Enigmatic Culprit

One rainy afternoon, She sat by the window, sipping chamomile tea. The pitter-patter of raindrops played a melancholic tune, and she leafed through old cookbooks. That's when she stumbled upon a chapter titled "Anemia: The Silent Thief."

"Anemia," she whispered, tracing the word with her fingertip. "A name that conceals both mystery and misery."

The pages revealed secrets—the kind that whispered in hushed tones, like ancient legends passed down through generations. Anemia wasn't a dragon to slay or a curse to break; it was a subtle thief, stealing vitality drop by drop. It thrived in shadows, camouflaged by everyday fatigue, pale skin, and breathlessness.

The Symphony of Blood

She delved deeper. She learned that anemia danced within our veins, orchestrating a symphony of blood cells. Iron, the conductor, wielded its baton, urging red blood cells to carry oxygen to every corner of our bodies. When iron faltered, the symphony turned discordant—a haunting melody of weakness and dizziness.

"But why?" She asked the raindrops, as if they held the answers. "Why does iron play hide-and-seek? Why do some notes falter while others soar?"

The Healing Cauldron

Determined, She brewed her own cauldron of knowledge. She stirred in dark leafy greens, lentils, and sunflower seeds—the magical ingredients that whispered promises of renewal. She sprinkled in vitamin C, like stardust, to unlock iron's hidden chambers. And she chanted incantations of balance—

pairing iron-rich foods with citrus companions.

"This," she declared, "is my potion against the silent thief."

Iron: The Silent Architect

The Oxygen Courier

Iron's primary duty is to escort oxygen. Picture a bustling airport terminal: red blood cells line up, passports stamped with iron's seal. These cells journey through your bloodstream, delivering life-sustaining oxygen to tissues, organs, and muscles. Without iron, this airport would be deserted, and the planes grounded.

Iron transforms food into energy. It's the alchemist in your metabolic laboratory, converting nutrients into ATP—the currency of vitality. When iron waltzes with other nutrients (like B vitamins), the dance floor lights up, and fatigue retreats.

Meet hemoglobin—the crimson conductor. Hemoglobin is a protein that cradles iron like a precious gem. Together, they form red blood cells— the maestros of oxygen transport. When iron orchestrates this symphony, you feel alive, vibrant, ready to conquer mountains (or at least climb a few flights of stairs).

The Immune Sentinel

The Immune Sentinel

Iron guards your immune fortress. White blood cells wield iron swords, defending against invaders. They patrol your body, ensuring harmony. When iron levels dip, these sentinels weaken, leaving your castle vulnerable.

The Brain's Muse

Iron whispers to your brain cells. It fuels cognition, memory, and creativity. Imagine iron as the ink in your mental quill, penning stories, solving puzzles, and composing sonnets. Without it, the library of your mind gathers dust.

Iron-Rich Foods: Your Treasure Chest

Now, let's explore the culinary map to replenish our iron reserves:

Leafy Greens: Spinach, kale, and Swiss chard—these verdant gems boast iron and vitamin C, a dynamic duo that enhances absorption.

Legumes Lentils, chickpeas, and black beans—these humble legumes pack a punch. They're like tiny iron-filled treasure chests buried in your pantry.

Whole Grains: Quinoa, brown rice, and oats—grains that whisper ancient secrets. Their iron content fuels your day like a sunrise over rolling hills.

Nuts and Seeds: Almonds, pumpkin seeds, and sunflower seeds—crunchy companions on your iron quest. They're the trail mix for your journey.

The Green Bounty: Leafy Greens

Spinach: This emerald superstar boasts iron, folate, and vitamin C. Imagine Popeye's biceps fueled by spinach—the same magic awaits you. Add it to salads, smoothies, or sauté it with garlic for a celestial side dish.

Kale: Kale dances in shades of green, its curly leaves like miniature forests. Iron, calcium, and antioxidants waltz within. Make kale chips, toss it in stir-fries, or blend it into pesto.

Swiss Chard: Picture vibrant rainbow stems—red, yellow, and pink—holding iron like precious gems. Swiss chard graces soups, stews, and frittatas. Its earthy flavor sings of health.

The Legume Symphony: Beans and Lentils

Lentils: These tiny legumes pack a punch. Red, green, or black—take your pick. Lentils are iron-rich and versatile. Simmer them into soups, fold them into curries, or create hearty salads.

Chickpeas: Hummus lovers, rejoice! Chickpeas are your allies. Their iron content harmonizes with fiber and protein. Roast them for crunchy snacks or toss them into Mediterranean bowls.

Black Beans: Midnight-hued and velvety, black beans offer iron, folate, and antioxidants. Mash them into burgers, layer them in enchiladas, or let them star in spicy chili.

Whole Grains

Quinoa: Ancient grains hold secrets. Quinoa, with its nutty flavor, is a complete protein and an iron powerhouse. Pilaf, salads, or breakfast bowls—quinoa adapts gracefully.

Brown Rice: Swap white rice for brown—the nutrient-rich sibling. Brown rice whispers tales of iron, magnesium, and fiber. Pair it with stir-fries or serve it alongside curries.

Oats: Morning magic lies in oats. Creamy porridge, overnight oats, or baked oatmeal—choose your adventure.

Iron and beta-glucans weave health into every spoonful.

The Nutty Serenade: Nuts and Seeds

Almonds: Almonds, like polished mahogany, harbor iron and vitamin E. Snack on them, sprinkle them over salads, or blend them into creamy almond butter.

Pumpkin Seeds: These tiny green warriors guard iron and zinc. Roast them with spices or scatter them atop soups. They're the crunchy knights of your plate.

Sunflower Seeds: Sunflowers turn their faces toward the sun, absorbing its energy. Their seeds gift you iron, selenium, and joy. Toss them into

granola or sprinkle them over avocado
toast.

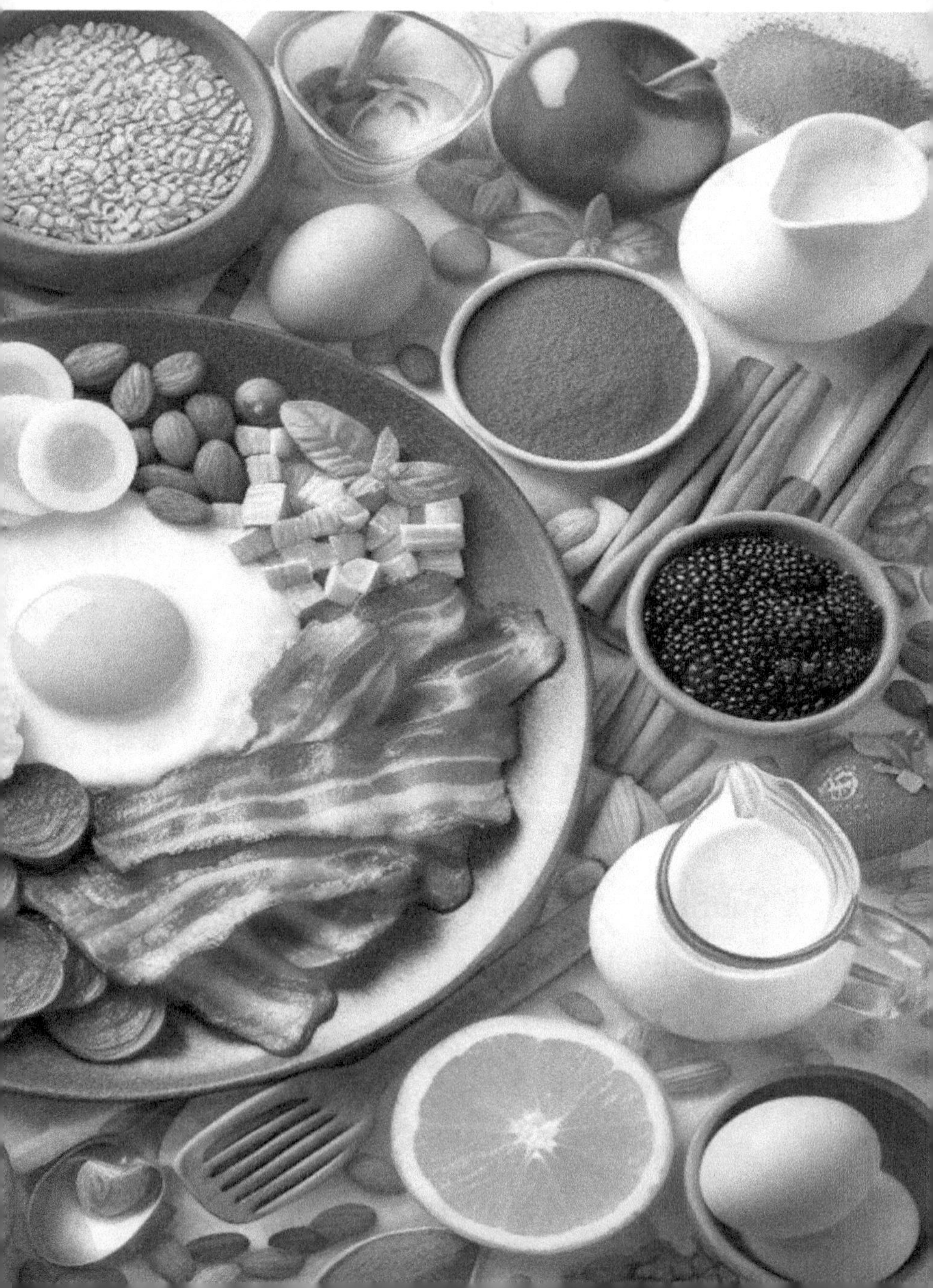

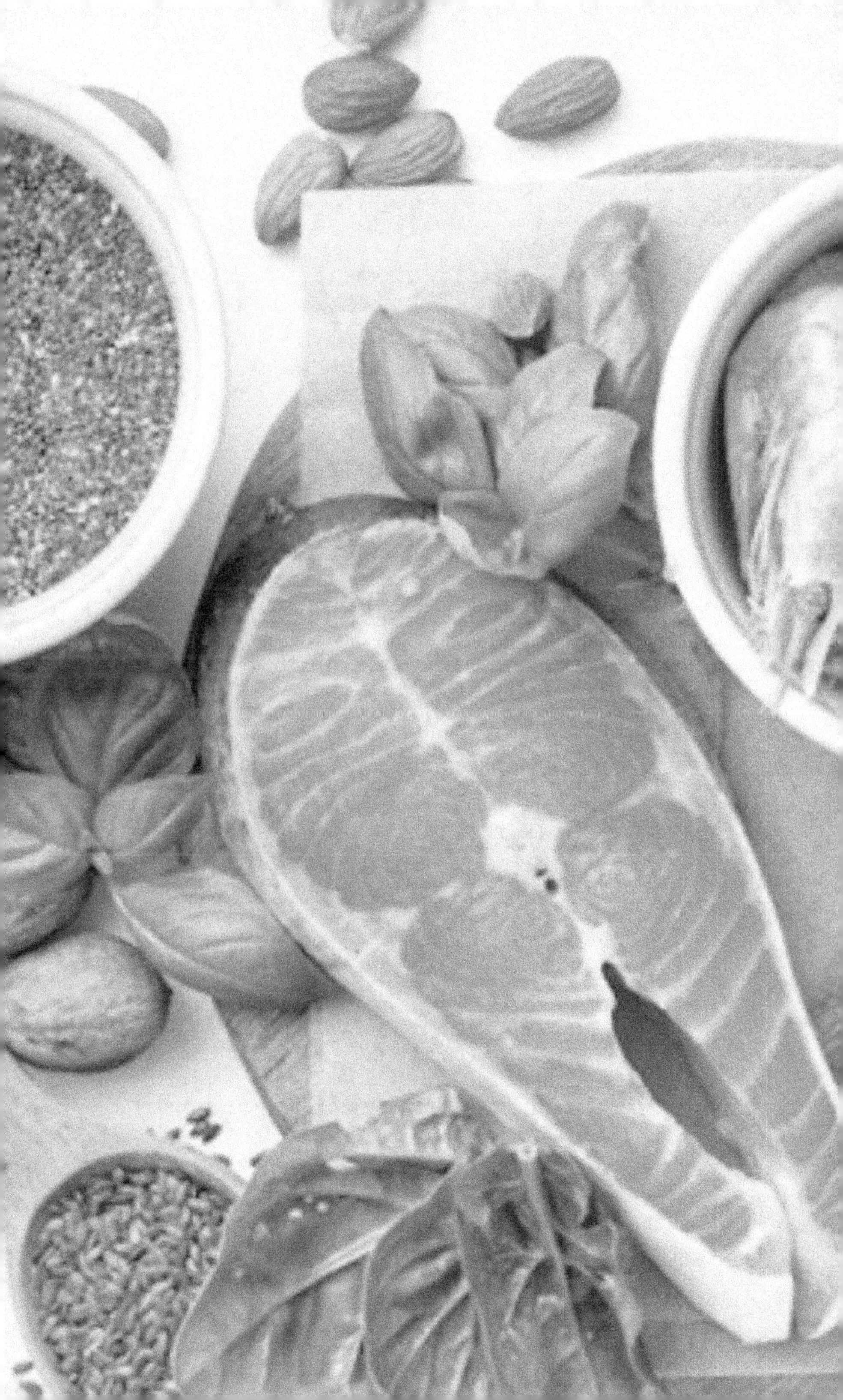

CHAPTER ONE

BREAKFAST RECIPES

Basil & Spinach Scramble

Ingredients (for 2 people):

- 2 tbsp olive oil
- 100g cherry tomatoes
- 4 eggs
- 60ml milk
- Handful of basil, chopped
- 200g baby spinach
- Salt and pepper

Instructions:

1. Heat olive oil in a non-stick pan.
2. Add cherry tomatoes and sauté until softened.

3. Whisk eggs with milk, basil, salt, and pepper.

4. Pour the egg mixture into the pan and scramble.

5. Add baby spinach and cook until wilted.

6. Serve hot with whole-grain toast.

Nutritional Information (per serving):

✓ Calories: 294

✓ Protein: 16g

✓ Carbs: 8g

✓ Fat: 24g

Fruit & Yogurt Smoothie

Ingredients:

● Greek yogurt

● Fruit juice (e.g., orange or pineapple)

- Frozen mixed berries (blueberries, strawberries, raspberries)

1. Blend Greek yogurt, fruit juice, and frozen berries until smooth.
2. Adjust consistency by adding more juice or yogurt.
3. Sip your refreshing and vitamin-rich smoothie.

- ✓ Calories: Varies based on ingredients
- ✓ Protein: Varies
- ✓ Carbs: Varies
- ✓ Fat: Varies

Peanut Butter & Chia Berry Jam English Muffin

Ingredients:

- Whole-grain English muffin
- Peanut butter
- Mixed berry jam (with chia seeds)

Instructions:

1. Toast the English muffin halves.
2. Spread peanut butter on one side and chia berry jam on the other.
3. Assemble and savor the omega-3 goodness.

Nutritional Information (per serving):

- ✓ Calories: Varies based on portion size
- ✓ Protein: Varies
- ✓ Carbs: Varies

- ✓ Fat: Varies

Spinach & Egg Scramble with Raspberries

Ingredients:

- Fresh spinach
- Eggs
- Whole-grain bread
- Raspberries

Instructions:

1. Sauté spinach until wilted.
2. Scramble eggs and fold in the spinach.
3. Serve with whole-grain toast and raspberries.

Nutritional Information (per serving):

- ✓ Calories: Varies based on portion size
- ✓ Protein: Varies
- ✓ Carbs: Varies
- ✓ Fat: Varies

Strawberry-Chocolate Smoothie

Ingredients:

- Frozen strawberries
- Cocoa powder
- Greek yogurt
- Almond milk

Instructions:

1. Blend strawberries, cocoa powder, Greek yogurt, and almond milk.
2. Satisfy your chocolate cravings guilt-free.

- ✓ Calories: Varies based on ingredients
- ✓ Protein: Varies
- ✓ Carbs: Varies
- ✓ Fat: Varies

Iron-Boosting Overnight Oats

Ingredients:

- 1/2 cup rolled oats
- 1 tablespoon chia seeds
- 1 cup almond milk (or any milk of your choice)
- 1 ripe banana, mashed
- 1 tablespoon honey or maple syrup
- A handful of sliced almonds

Instructions:

1. In a jar, combine rolled oats, chia seeds, mashed banana, and almond milk.

2. Stir well and refrigerate overnight.

3. In the morning, drizzle with honey or maple syrup and top with sliced almonds.

- ✓ Calories: 350
- ✓ Protein: 8g
- ✓ Carbs: 55g
- ✓ Fat: 12g

Iron-Infused Chia Pudding

Ingredients:

- 2 tablespoons chia seeds
- 1 cup coconut milk (or any milk)
- 1 teaspoon cocoa powder

- 1 tablespoon almond butter
- Sliced strawberries for topping

1. Mix chia seeds, coconut milk, cocoa powder, and almond butter in a bowl.
2. Refrigerate for at least 2 hours (or overnight) until it thickens.
3. Serve chilled, topped with sliced strawberries.

- ✓ Calories: 280
- ✓ Protein: 6g
- ✓ Carbs: 20g
- ✓ Fat: 20g

Iron-Rich Quinoa Breakfast Bowl

Ingredients:

- 1/2 cup cooked quinoa
- 1 tablespoon pumpkin seeds
- 1 tablespoon dried cranberries
- Sliced kiwi or orange segments
- A drizzle of honey

Instructions:

1. Mix cooked quinoa with pumpkin seeds and dried cranberries.
2. Top with sliced kiwi or orange segments.
3. Drizzle with honey for natural sweetness.

Nutritional Information (per serving):

✓ Calories: 250

- ✓ Protein: 6g

- ✓ Carbs: 45g

- ✓ Fat: 5g

Iron-Packed Green Smoothie

Ingredients:

- Handful of spinach

- 1 ripe banana

- 1 tablespoon almond butter

- 1 cup almond milk

- Ice cubes

Instructions:

1. Blend spinach, banana, almond butter, and almond milk until smooth.

2. Add ice cubes and blend again.

3. Sip your iron-rich green goodness.

- ✓ Calories: 220
- ✓ Protein: 5g
- ✓ Carbs: 35g
- ✓ Fat: 8g

Iron-Boosting Berry Parfait

Ingredients:

- Greek yogurt
- Mixed berries (blueberries, raspberries, strawberries)
- Granola (choose a fortified one for extra iron)
- A sprinkle of flaxseeds

Instructions:

1. Layer Greek yogurt, mixed berries, and granola in a glass.
2. Repeat the layers.

3. Top with flax-seeds for added nutrition.

- ✓ Calories: 300
- ✓ Protein: 15g
- ✓ Carbs: 45g
- ✓ Fat: 8g

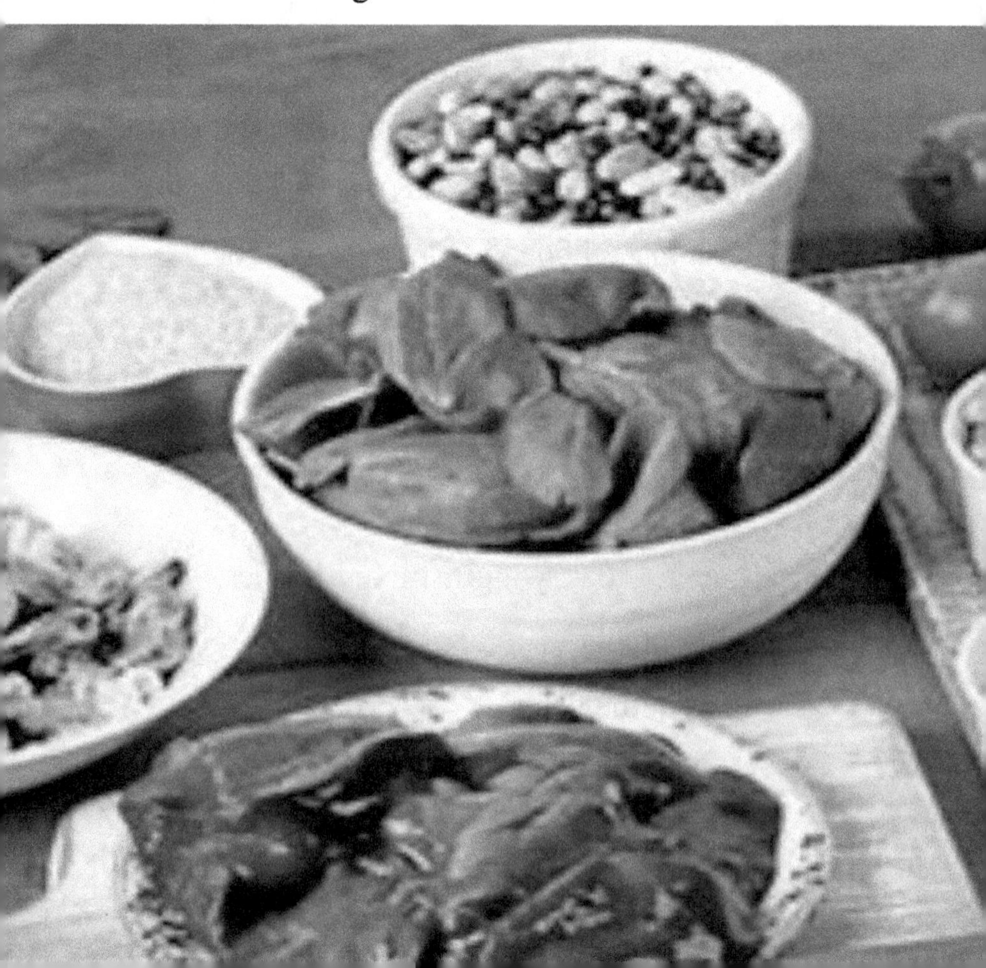

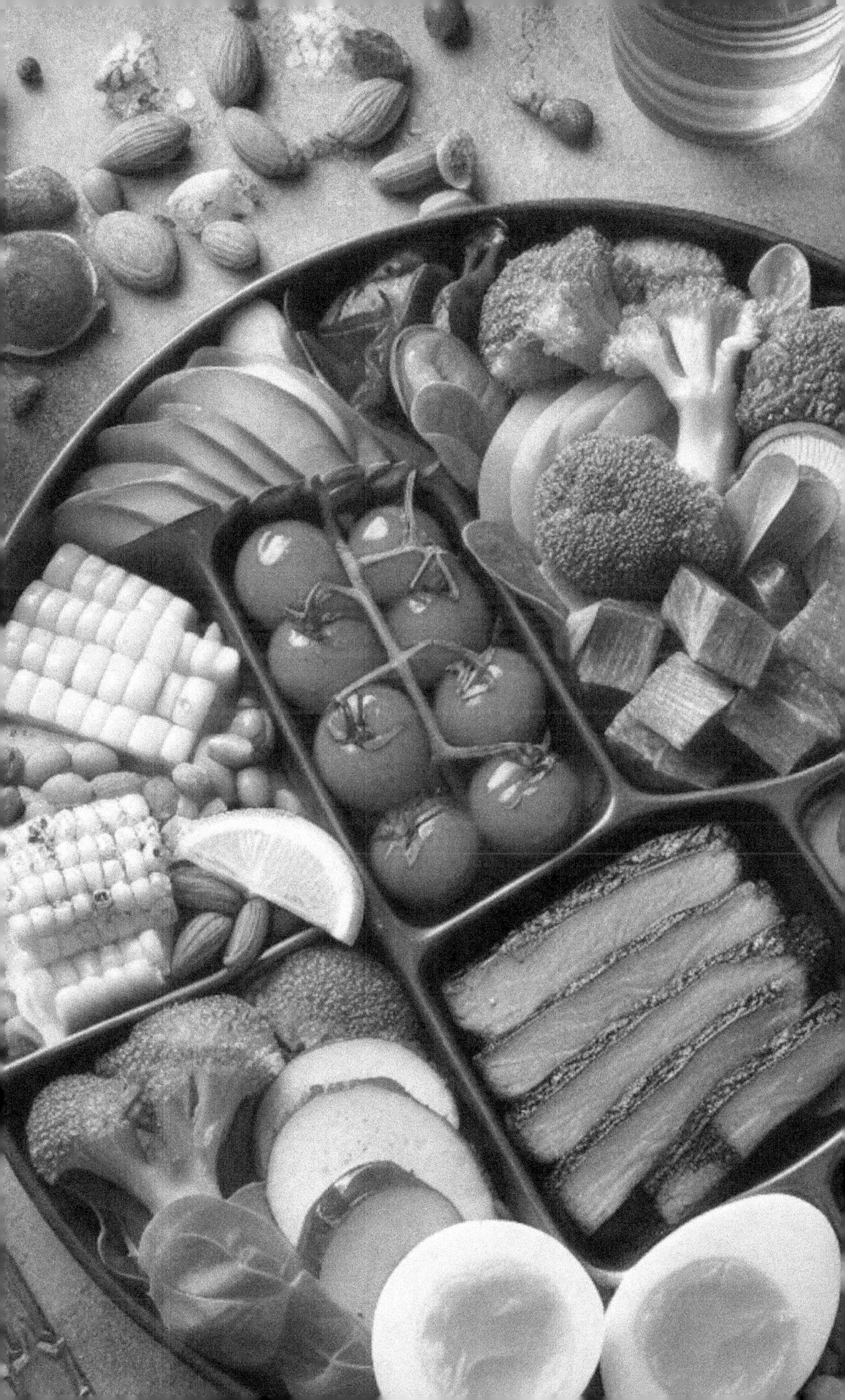

CHAPTER TWO

LUNCH AND DINNER IDEAS

Iron-Boosting Lentil Soup

Ingredients (serves 4):

- 1 cup green or brown lentils
- 1 onion, chopped
- 2 carrots, diced
- 2 celery stalks, chopped
- 4 cups vegetable broth
- 1 teaspoon cumin
- Salt and pepper to taste
- Fresh parsley for garnish

Instructions:

1. Rinse lentils and set aside.
2. Sauté onion, carrots, and celery in a pot until softened.

3. Add lentils, vegetable broth, cumin, salt, and pepper.

4. Simmer for 30 minutes or until lentils are tender.

5. Garnish with fresh parsley and serve.

- ✓ Calories: 250
- ✓ Protein: 15g
- ✓ Carbs: 45g
- ✓ Fat: 2g

Spinach and Chickpea Salad

Ingredients (serves 2):

- 2 cups fresh spinach
- 1 cup canned chickpeas, drained
- 1 red bell pepper, sliced
- 1 cucumber, diced

- Feta cheese (optional)
- Lemon-tahini dressing

1. Toss spinach, chickpeas, bell pepper, and cucumber in a bowl.
2. Drizzle with lemon-tahini dressing.
3. Top with crumbled feta if desired.

- ✓ Calories: 280
- ✓ Protein: 12g
- ✓ Carbs: 40g
- ✓ Fat: 10g

Quinoa-Stuffed Bell Peppers

- 4 bell peppers (any color)
- 1 cup cooked quinoa

- 1 cup black beans (canned or cooked)
- 1 cup diced tomatoes
- 1 teaspoon cumin
- Salt and pepper to taste
- Fresh cilantro for garnish

Instructions:

1. Preheat oven to 375°F (190°C).
2. Cut tops off bell peppers and remove seeds.
3. Mix cooked quinoa, black beans, diced tomatoes, cumin, salt, and pepper.
4. Stuff peppers with quinoa mixture.
5. Bake for 25-30 minutes.
6. Garnish with fresh cilantro.

Nutritional Information (per serving):

✓ Calories: 220

- ✓ Protein: 10g
- ✓ Carbs: 40g
- ✓ Fat: 2g

Salmon with Lemon-Dill Sauce

Ingredients (serves 2):

- 2 salmon fillets
- Juice of 1 lemon
- Fresh dill, chopped
- Salt and pepper
- Steamed asparagus or green beans

Instructions:

1. Season salmon with lemon juice, dill, salt, and pepper.
2. Grill or bake salmon until cooked.
3. Serve with steamed asparagus or green beans.

Nutritional Information (per serving):

- ✓ Calories: 300
- ✓ Protein: 30g
- ✓ Carbs: 5g
- ✓ Fat: 18g

Iron-Rich Stir-Fry

Ingredients (serves 4):

- 1 cup broccoli florets
- 1 red bell pepper, sliced
- 1 cup sliced mushrooms
- 1 cup tofu or tempeh, cubed
- 2 tablespoons soy sauce
- 1 tablespoon sesame oil
- Brown rice or quinoa

1. Sauté broccoli, bell pepper, mushrooms, and tofu/tempeh in sesame oil.
2. Add soy sauce and stir-fry until veggies are tender.
3. Serve over brown rice or quinoa.

- ✓ Calories: 280
- ✓ Protein: 20g
- ✓ Carbs: 30g
- ✓ Fat: 10g

Iron-Boosting Lentil Soup

- 1 cup green or brown lentils
- 1 onion, chopped
- 2 carrots, diced
- 2 celery stalks, chopped

- 4 cups vegetable broth

- 1 teaspoon cumin

- Salt and pepper to taste

- Fresh parsley for garnish

Instructions:

1. Rinse lentils and set aside.

2. Sauté onion, carrots, and celery in a pot until softened.

3. Add lentils, vegetable broth, cumin, salt, and pepper.

4. Simmer for 30 minutes or until lentils are tender.

5. Garnish with fresh parsley and serve.

Nutritional Information (per serving):

✓ Calories: 250

- ✓ Protein: 15g
- ✓ Carbs: 45g
- ✓ Fat: 2g

Spinach and Chickpea Salad

Ingredients (serves 2):

- 2 cups fresh spinach
- 1 cup canned chickpeas, drained
- 1 red bell pepper, sliced
- 1 cucumber, diced
- Feta cheese (optional)
- Lemon-tahini dressing

Instructions:

1. Toss spinach, chickpeas, bell pepper, and cucumber in a bowl.
2. Drizzle with lemon-tahini dressing.
3. Top with crumbled feta if desired.

- ✓ Calories: 280
- ✓ Protein: 12g
- ✓ Carbs: 40g
- ✓ Fat: 10g

Quinoa-Stuffed Bell Peppers

Ingredients (serves 4):

- 4 bell peppers (any color)
- 1 cup cooked quinoa
- 1 cup black beans (canned or cooked)
- 1 cup diced tomatoes
- 1 teaspoon cumin
- Salt and pepper to taste
- Fresh cilantro for garnish

1. Preheat oven to 375°F (190°C).

2. Cut tops off bell peppers and remove seeds.

3. Mix cooked quinoa, black beans, diced tomatoes, cumin, salt, and pepper.

4. Stuff peppers with quinoa mixture.

5. Bake for 25-30 minutes.

6. Garnish with fresh cilantro.

Nutritional Information (per serving):

- ✓ Calories: 220
- ✓ Protein: 10g
- ✓ Carbs: 40g
- ✓ Fat: 2g

Salmon with Lemon-Dill Sauce

Ingredients (serves 2):

- 2 salmon fillets
- Juice of 1 lemon
- Fresh dill, chopped
- Salt and pepper
- Steamed asparagus or green beans

Instructions:

1. Season salmon with lemon juice, dill, salt, and pepper.
2. Grill or bake salmon until cooked.
3. Serve with steamed asparagus or green beans.

Nutritional Information (per serving):

- ✓ Calories: 300
- ✓ Protein: 30g
- ✓ Carbs: 5g

✓ Fat: 18g

Iron-Rich Stir-Fry

Ingredients (serves 4):

- 1 cup broccoli florets
- 1 red bell pepper, sliced
- 1 cup sliced mushrooms
- 1 cup tofu or tempeh, cubed
- 2 tablespoons soy sauce
- 1 tablespoon sesame oil
- Brown rice or quinoa

Instructions:

1. Sauté broccoli, bell pepper, mushrooms, and tofu/tempeh in sesame oil.
2. Add soy sauce and stir-fry until veggies are tender.
3. Serve over brown rice or quinoa.

Nutritional Information (per serving):

- ✓ Calories: 280
- ✓ Protein: 20g
- ✓ Carbs: 30g
- ✓ Fat: 10g

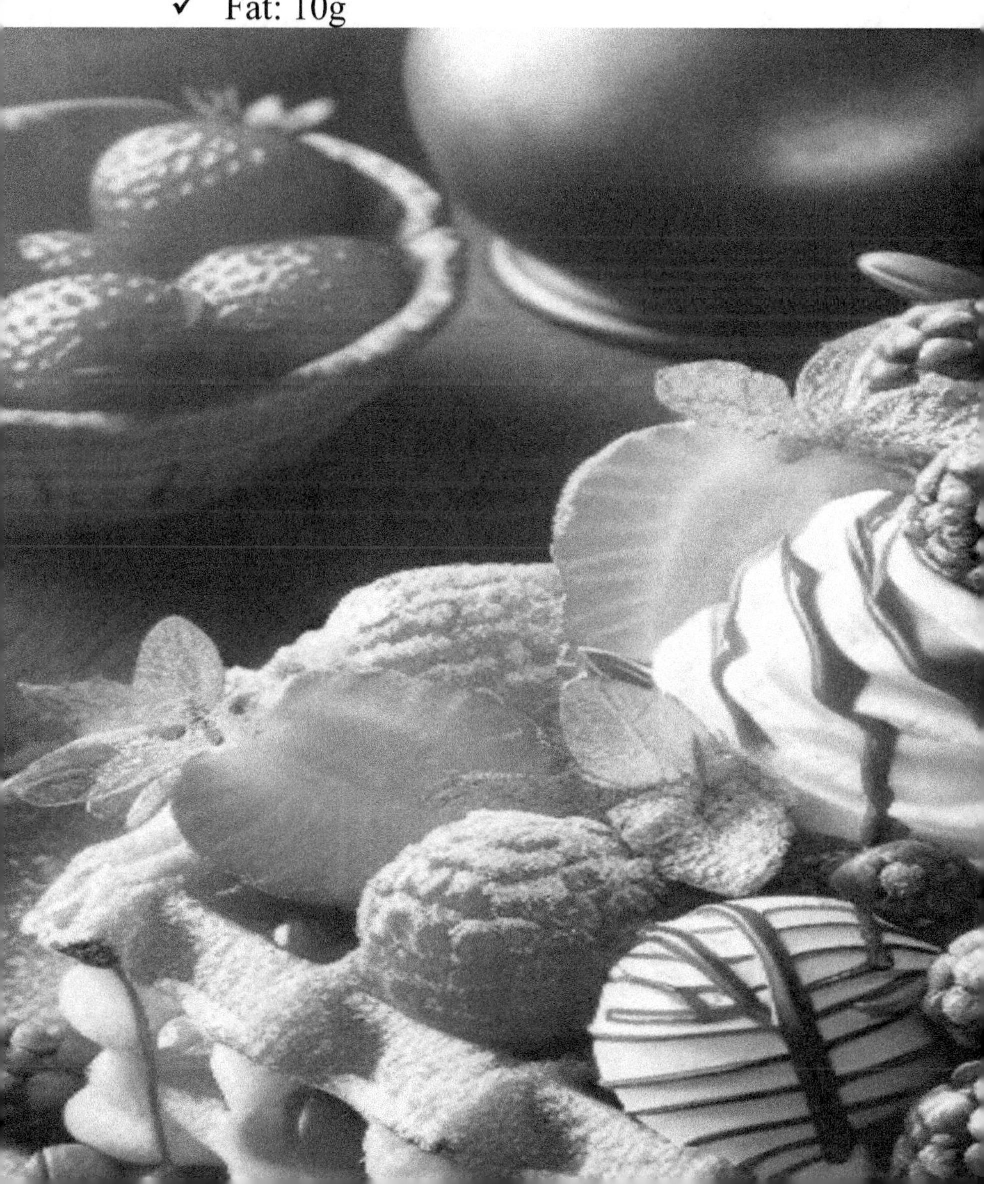

CHAPTER THREE

DELICIOUS DESSERTS

Dark Chocolate-Dipped Strawberries

Ingredients (serves 4):

- 1 cup fresh strawberries
- 3 oz dark chocolate (70% cocoa or higher)
- Crushed almonds or pistachios for topping

Instructions:

1. Melt dark chocolate in a microwave-safe bowl.
2. Dip each strawberry into the melted chocolate.

3. Place on parchment paper and sprinkle with crushed nuts.

4. Let them cool and harden.

- ✓ Calories: 120
- ✓ Protein: 2g
- ✓ Carbs: 15g
- ✓ Fat: 7g

Iron-Infused Chia Seed Pudding

Ingredients (serves 2):

- 1/4 cup chia seeds
- 1 cup almond milk
- 1 tablespoon unsweetened cocoa powder
- 1 tablespoon maple syrup
- Sliced bananas for topping

Instructions:

Instructions:

1. Mix chia seeds, almond milk, cocoa powder, and maple syrup.
2. Refrigerate for at least 2 hours (or overnight) until thickened.
3. Layer with sliced bananas.

Nutritional Information (per serving):

- ✓ Calories: 180
- ✓ Protein: 4g
- ✓ Carbs: 25g
- ✓ Fat: 8g

Baked Apples with Cinnamon and Walnuts

Ingredients (serves 4):

- 4 medium apples (such as Granny Smith)
- 1 teaspoon cinnamon

- 1/4 cup chopped walnuts
- 1 tablespoon honey

1. Preheat oven to 375°F (190°C).
2. Core the apples and place them in a baking dish.
3. Sprinkle with cinnamon and stuff with chopped walnuts.
4. Drizzle with honey.
5. Bake for 30-35 minutes until tender.
6. Serve warm.

Nutritional Information (per serving):

- ✓ Calories: 150
- ✓ Protein: 2g
- ✓ Carbs: 30g
- ✓ Fat: 4g

Berry Parfait with Greek Yogurt

Ingredients (serves 2):

- 1 cup Greek yogurt
- 1 cup mixed berries (blueberries, raspberries, strawberries)
- 1 tablespoon honey
- Granola for crunch

Instructions:

1. Layer Greek yogurt, mixed berries, and granola in glasses.
2. Drizzle with honey.

A protein-packed and antioxidant-rich dessert!

Nutritional Information (per serving):

- ✓ Calories: 200
- ✓ Protein: 15g
- ✓ Carbs: 30g

✓ Fat: 3g

Iron-Boosting Chocolate Avocado Mousse

Ingredients (serves 2):

- 1 ripe avocado
- 2 tablespoons unsweetened cocoa powder
- 2 tablespoons maple syrup
- A pinch of salt
- Sliced almonds for garnish

Instructions:

1. Blend avocado, cocoa powder, maple syrup, and salt until smooth.
2. Chill in the refrigerator.
3. Top with sliced almonds before serving.

- ✓ Calories: 220
- ✓ Protein: 3g
- ✓ Carbs: 20g
- ✓ Fat: 15g

Iron-Boosting Lentil Soup

Ingredients (serves 4):

- 1 cup green or brown lentils
- 1 onion, chopped
- 2 carrots, diced
- 2 celery stalks, chopped
- 4 cups vegetable broth
- 1 teaspoon cumin
- Salt and pepper to taste
- Fresh parsley for garnish

Instructions:

1. Rinse lentils and set aside.

2. Sauté onion, carrots, and celery in a pot until softened.

3. Add lentils, vegetable broth, cumin, salt, and pepper.

4. Simmer for 30 minutes or until lentils are tender.

5. Garnish with fresh parsley and serve.

Nutritional Information (per serving):

✓ Calories: 250

✓ Protein: 15g

✓ Carbs: 45g

✓ Fat: 2g

Spinach and Chickpea Salad

Ingredients (serves 2):

1. 2 cups fresh spinach

2. 1 cup canned chickpeas, drained

3. 1 red bell pepper, sliced

4. 1 cucumber, diced

5. Feta cheese (optional)

6. Lemon-tahini dressing

7. Instructions:

8. Toss spinach, chickpeas, bell pepper, and cucumber in a bowl.

9. Drizzle with lemon-tahini dressing.

10. Top with crumbled feta if desired.

Nutritional Information (per serving):

- ✓ Calories: 280
- ✓ Protein: 12g
- ✓ Carbs: 40g
- ✓ Fat: 10g

Quinoa-Stuffed Bell Peppers

Ingredients (serves 4):

- 4 bell peppers (any color)

- 1 cup cooked quinoa
- 1 cup black beans (canned or cooked)
- 1 cup diced tomatoes
- 1 teaspoon cumin
- Salt and pepper to taste
- Fresh cilantro for garnish

Instructions:

1. Preheat oven to 375°F (190°C).
2. Cut tops off bell peppers and remove seeds.
3. Mix cooked quinoa, black beans, diced tomatoes, cumin, salt, and pepper.
4. Stuff peppers with quinoa mixture.
5. Bake for 25-30 minutes.
6. Garnish with fresh cilantro.

Nutritional Information (per serving):

- ✓ Calories: 220
- ✓ Protein: 10g
- ✓ Carbs: 40g
- ✓ Fat: 2g

Salmon with Lemon-Dill Sauce

Ingredients (serves 2):

- 2 salmon fillets
- Juice of 1 lemon
- Fresh dill, chopped
- Salt and pepper
- Steamed asparagus or green beans

Instructions:

1. Season salmon with lemon juice, dill, salt, and pepper.
2. Grill or bake salmon until cooked.

3. Serve with steamed asparagus or
   green beans.

✓ Calories: 300

✓ Protein: 30g

✓ Carbs: 5g

✓ Fat: 18g

Iron-Rich Stir-Fry

Ingredients (serves 4):

- 1 cup broccoli florets
- 1 red bell pepper, sliced
- 1 cup sliced mushrooms
- 1 cup tofu or tempeh, cubed
- 2 tablespoons soy sauce
- 1 tablespoon sesame oil
- Brown rice or quinoa

1. Sauté broccoli, bell pepper, mushrooms, and tofu/tempeh in sesame oil.

2. Add soy sauce and stir-fry until veggies are tender.

3. Serve over brown rice or quinoa.

Nutritional Information (per serving):

✓ Calories: 280

✓ Protein: 20g

✓ Carbs: 30g

✓ Fat: 10g

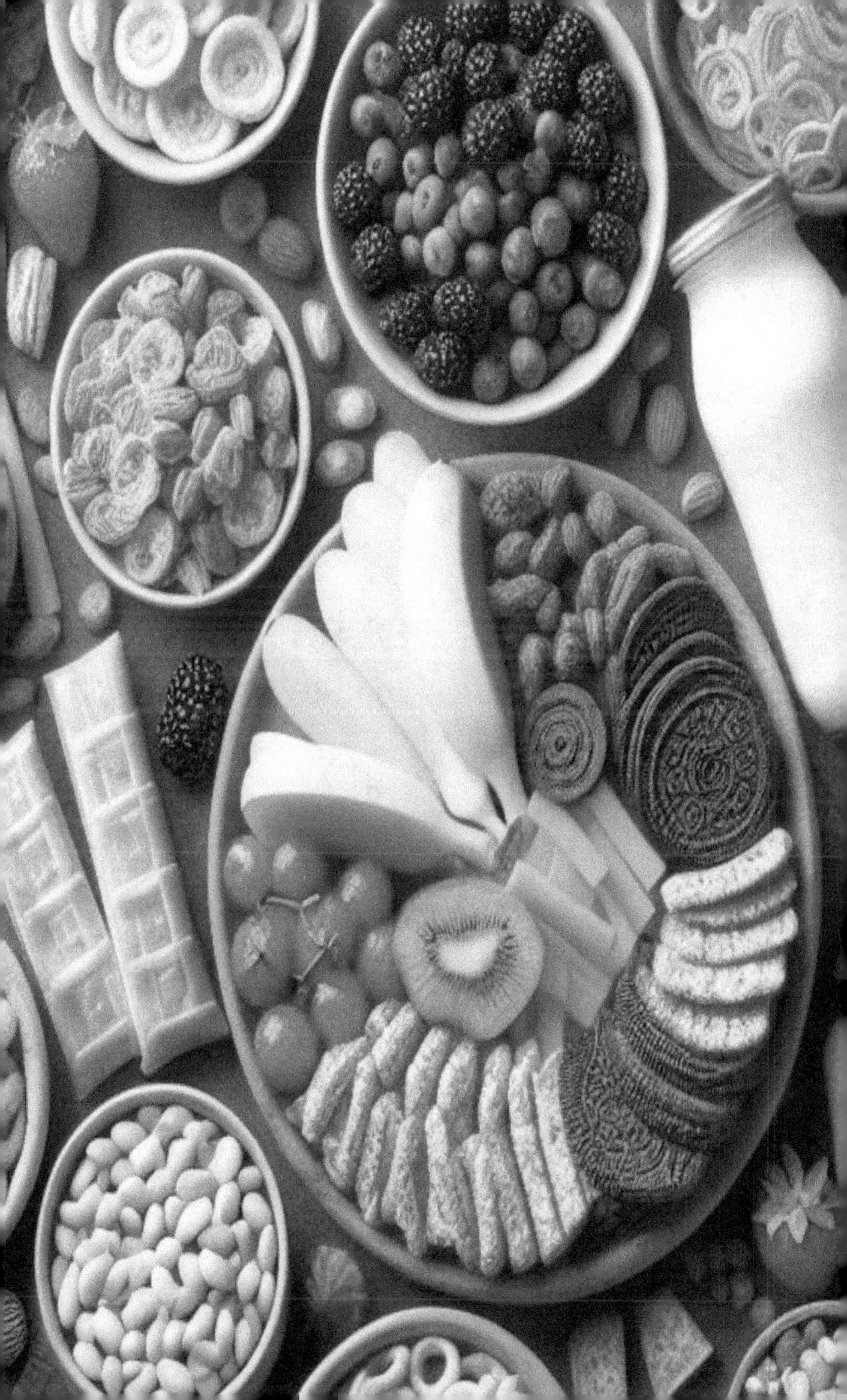

CHAPTER FOUR
SNACKS AND SIDES

Iron-Infused Guacamole

Ingredients (serves 4):

- 2 ripe avocados
- Juice of 1 lime
- 1 clove garlic, minced
- 1 small red onion, finely chopped
- 1 tomato, diced
- Fresh cilantro, chopped
- Salt and pepper to taste

Instructions:

1. Mash avocados in a bowl.
2. Add lime juice, minced garlic, chopped onion, diced tomato, and cilantro.
3. Season with salt and pepper.

4. Serve with whole-grain tortilla chips or carrot sticks.

Nutritional Information (per serving):

✓ Calories: 180

✓ Protein: 2g

✓ Carbs: 12g

✓ Fat: 15g

Roasted Beet Hummus

Ingredients (serves 4):

- 2 medium beets, roasted and peeled
- 1 can (15 oz) chickpeas, drained and rinsed
- 2 tablespoons tahini
- Juice of 1 lemon
- 1 clove garlic
- Salt and cumin to taste
- Olive oil for drizzling

1. Blend roasted beets, chickpeas, tahini, lemon juice, garlic, salt, and cumin in a food processor.
2. Drizzle with olive oil before serving.
3. Enjoy with whole-grain pita bread or veggie sticks.

Nutritional Information (per serving):

- ✓ Calories: 160
- ✓ Protein: 6g
- ✓ Carbs: 20g
- ✓ Fat: 7g

Kale and Quinoa Salad

Ingredients (serves 2):

- 2 cups kale, chopped
- 1 cup cooked quinoa
- 1/2 cup pomegranate arils

- 1/4 cup crumbled feta cheese
- 2 tablespoons balsamic vinaigrette

Instructions:

1. Massage kale with balsamic vinaigrette to soften.
2. Mix with cooked quinoa, pomegranate arils, and crumbled feta.

Nutritional Information (per serving):

- ✓ Calories: 220
- ✓ Protein: 8g
- ✓ Carbs: 30g
- ✓ Fat: 8g

Sweet Potato Fries

Ingredients (serves 4):

- 2 large sweet potatoes, cut into fries

- 1 tablespoon olive oil
- Paprika, garlic powder, and salt to taste

Instructions:

1. Toss sweet potato fries with olive oil and seasonings.
2. Bake at 400°F (200°C) for 25-30 minutes.

Crispy and iron-rich!

Nutritional Information (per serving):

- ✓ Calories: 150
- ✓ Protein: 2g
- ✓ Carbs: 30g
- ✓ Fat: 3g

Edamame Salad

- 1 cup cooked edamame (soybeans)
- 1 cucumber, diced
- 1 red bell pepper, sliced
- Fresh mint leaves, chopped
- Lime juice and sesame seeds for dressing

1. Mix cooked edamame, cucumber, bell pepper, and mint.
2. Drizzle with lime juice and sprinkle sesame seeds.

A refreshing and protein-packed side!

- ✓ Calories: 180
- ✓ Protein: 12g

- ✓ Carbs: 20g
- ✓ Fat: 7g

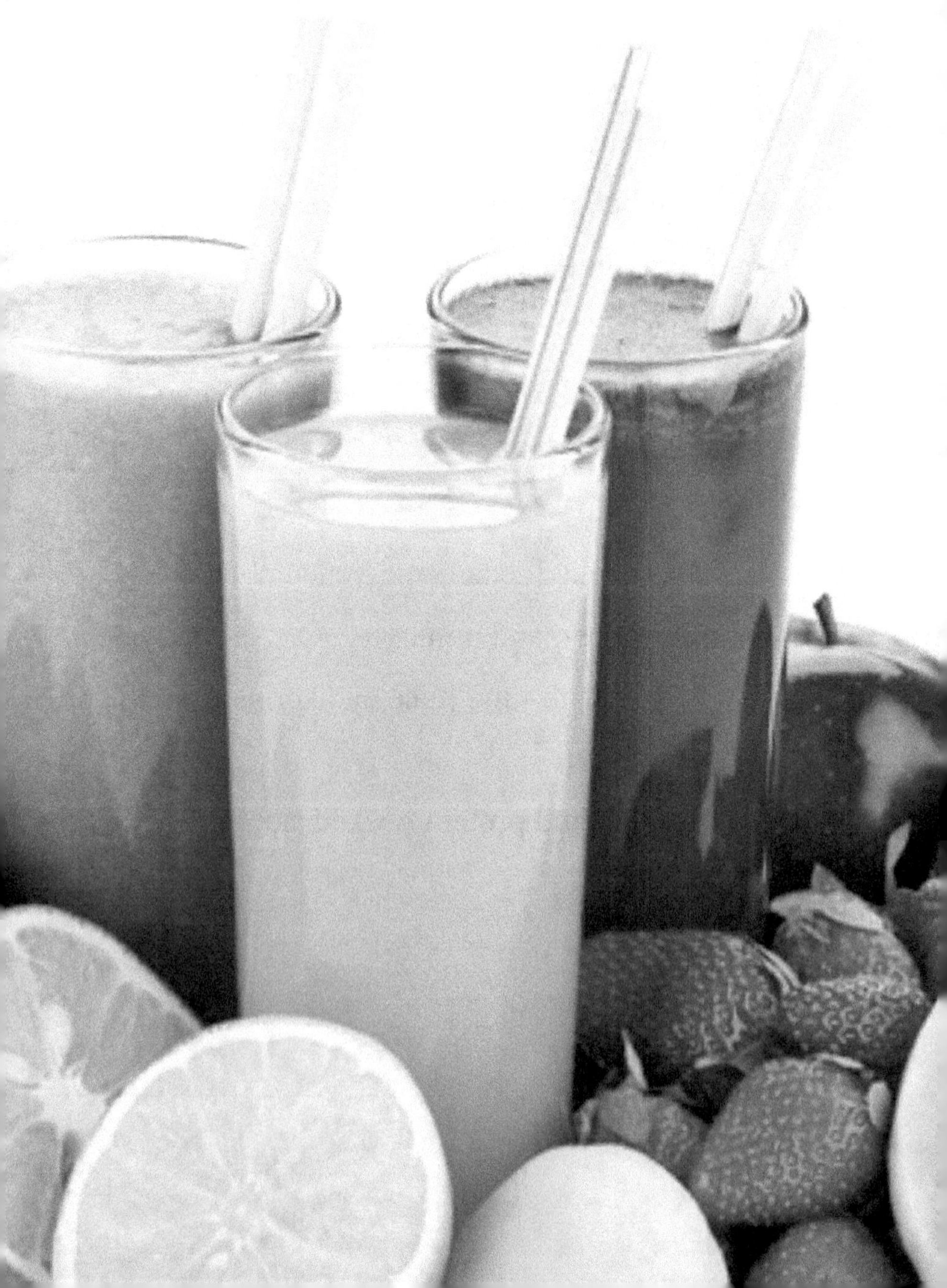

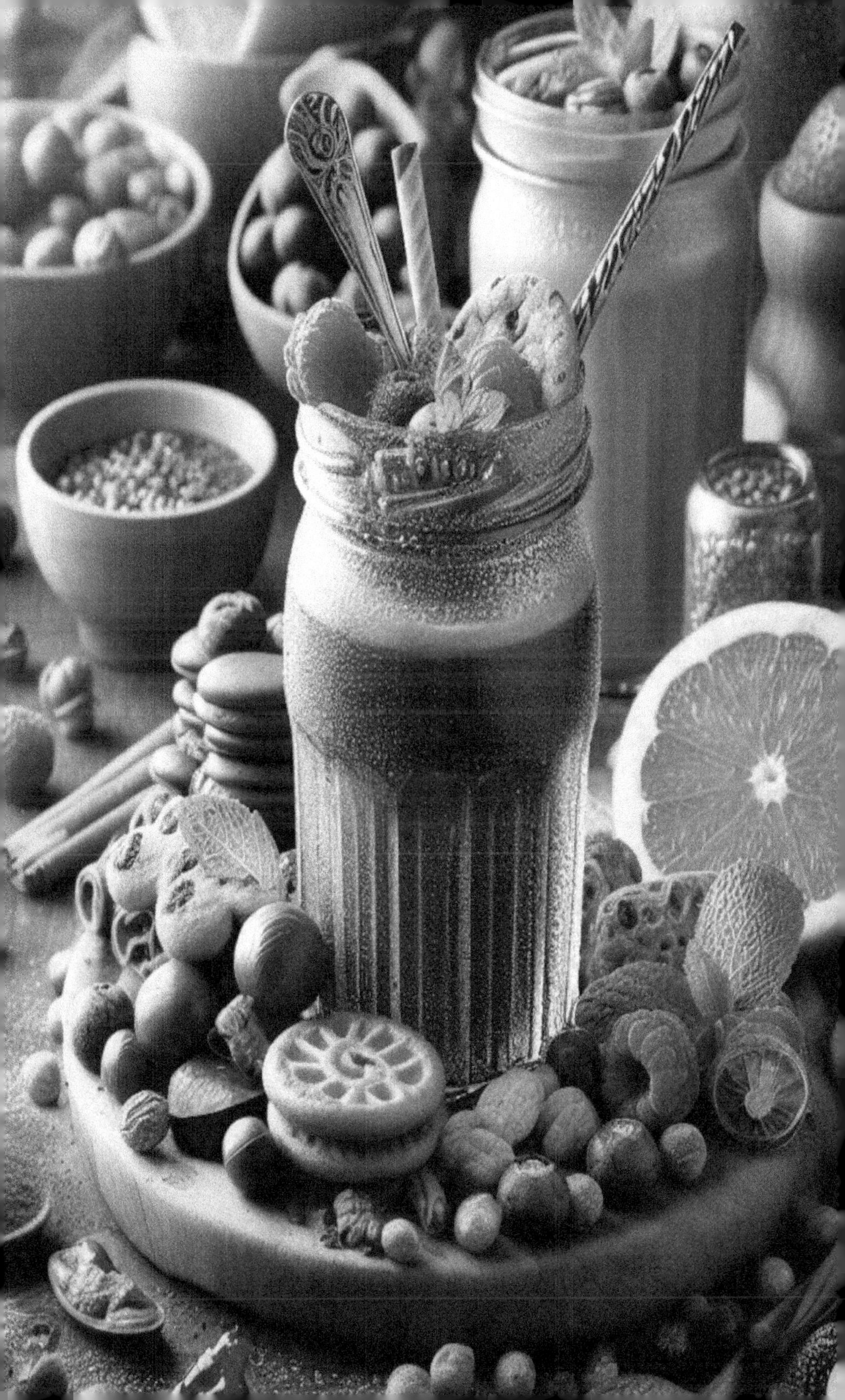

CHAPTER FIVE
BEVERAGES

Iron-Infused Green Smoothie

Ingredients (serves 2):

- 2 cups fresh spinach
- 1 ripe banana
- 1 cup unsweetened almond milk
- 1 tablespoon almond butter
- A handful of ice cubes

Instructions:

1. Blend spinach, banana, almond milk, and almond butter until smooth.
2. Add ice cubes and blend again.
3. Pour into glasses and enjoy your iron-packed green goodness!

- ✓ Calories: 150
- ✓ Protein: 5g
- ✓ Carbs: 20g
- ✓ Fat: 7g

Beetroot and Orange Juice

Ingredients (serves 2):

- 2 medium beets, peeled and chopped
- Juice of 4 oranges
- 1 teaspoon honey (optional)

Instructions:

- Juice the oranges and set aside.
- Blend the chopped beets with a little water until smooth.
- Mix the beetroot puree with orange juice.

- Add honey if desired.

Serve chilled for a refreshing and iron-rich drink!

- ✓ Calories: 120
- ✓ Protein: 2g
- ✓ Carbs: 28g
- ✓ Fat: 0g

Prune and Ginger Tea

Ingredients (serves 1):

- 3 dried prunes
- 1-inch fresh ginger, sliced
- 1 cup boiling water
- A squeeze of lemon (optional)

Instructions:

1. Place prunes and ginger in a teapot.

2. Pour boiling water over them and steep for 5-10 minutes.

3. Strain and serve warm.

Prunes are naturally high in iron!

Nutritional Information (per serving):

✓ Calories: 30

✓ Protein: 0g

✓ Carbs: 8g

✓ Fat: 0g

Kiwi and Spinach Smoothie

Ingredients (serves 2):

● 2 ripe kiwis, peeled and chopped

● 2 cups fresh spinach

● 1 cup coconut water

● A dash of lime juice

1. Blend kiwi, spinach, and coconut water until smooth.
2. Add lime juice for extra flavor.

A vitamin C-rich and iron-boosting drink!

- ✓ Calories: 80
- ✓ Protein: 2g
- ✓ Carbs: 18g
- ✓ Fat: 0g

Turmeric Golden Milk

- 1 cup unsweetened almond milk
- 1/2 teaspoon ground turmeric
- A pinch of black pepper
- A dash of honey (optional)

1. Heat almond milk in a saucepan.

2. Add turmeric and black pepper.

3. Whisk well and simmer for 5 minutes.

4. Sweeten with honey if desired.

Turmeric is anti-inflammatory and aids iron absorption!

✓ Calories: 40

✓ Protein: 1g

✓ Carbs: 6g

✓ Fat: 2g

Iron-Boosting Lentil Soup

● 1 cup green or brown lentils

● 1 onion, chopped

- 2 carrots, diced
- 2 celery stalks, chopped
- 4 cups vegetable broth
- 1 teaspoon cumin
- Salt and pepper to taste
- Fresh parsley for garnish

Instructions:

1. Rinse lentils and set aside.
2. Sauté onion, carrots, and celery in a pot until softened.
3. Add lentils, vegetable broth, cumin, salt, and pepper.
4. Simmer for 30 minutes or until lentils are tender.
5. Garnish with fresh parsley and serve.

- ✓ Calories: 250
- ✓ Protein: 15g
- ✓ Carbs: 45g
- ✓ Fat: 2g

Spinach and Chickpea Salad

Ingredients (serves 2):

- 2 cups fresh spinach
- 1 cup canned chickpeas, drained
- 1 red bell pepper, sliced
- 1 cucumber, diced
- Feta cheese (optional)
- Lemon-tahini dressing

Instructions:

1. Toss spinach, chickpeas, bell pepper, and cucumber in a bowl.
2. Drizzle with lemon-tahini dressing.

3. Top with crumbled feta if desired.

- ✓ Calories: 280
- ✓ Protein: 12g
- ✓ Carbs: 40g
- ✓ Fat: 10g

Quinoa-Stuffed Bell Peppers

Ingredients (serves 4):

- 4 bell peppers (any color)
- 1 cup cooked quinoa
- 1 cup black beans (canned or cooked)
- 1 cup diced tomatoes
- 1 teaspoon cumin
- Salt and pepper to taste
- Fresh cilantro for garnish

1. Preheat oven to 375°F (190°C).

2. Cut tops off bell peppers and remove seeds.

3. Mix cooked quinoa, black beans, diced tomatoes, cumin, salt, and pepper.

4. Stuff peppers with quinoa mixture.

5. Bake for 25-30 minutes.

6. Garnish with fresh cilantro.

Nutritional Information (per serving):

✓ Calories: 220

✓ Protein: 10g

✓ Carbs: 40g

✓ Fat: 2g

Salmon with Lemon-Dill Sauce

Ingredients (serves 2):

- 2 salmon fillets
- Juice of 1 lemon
- Fresh dill, chopped
- Salt and pepper
- Steamed asparagus or green beans

Instructions:

1. Season salmon with lemon juice, dill, salt, and pepper.
2. Grill or bake salmon until cooked.
3. Serve with steamed asparagus or green beans.

Nutritional Information (per serving):

- Calories: 300
- Protein: 30g
- Carbs: 5g
- Fat: 18g

Iron-Rich Stir-Fry

Ingredients (serves 4):

- 1 cup broccoli florets
- 1 red bell pepper, sliced
- 1 cup sliced mushrooms
- 1 cup tofu or tempeh, cubed
- 2 tablespoons soy sauce
- 1 tablespoon sesame oil
- Brown rice or quinoa

Instructions:

1. Sauté broccoli, bell pepper, mushrooms, and tofu/tempeh in sesame oil.
2. Add soy sauce and stir-fry until veggies are tender.
3. Serve over brown rice or quinoa.

- ✓ Calories: 280
- ✓ Protein: 20g
- ✓ Carbs: 30g
- ✓ Fat: 10g

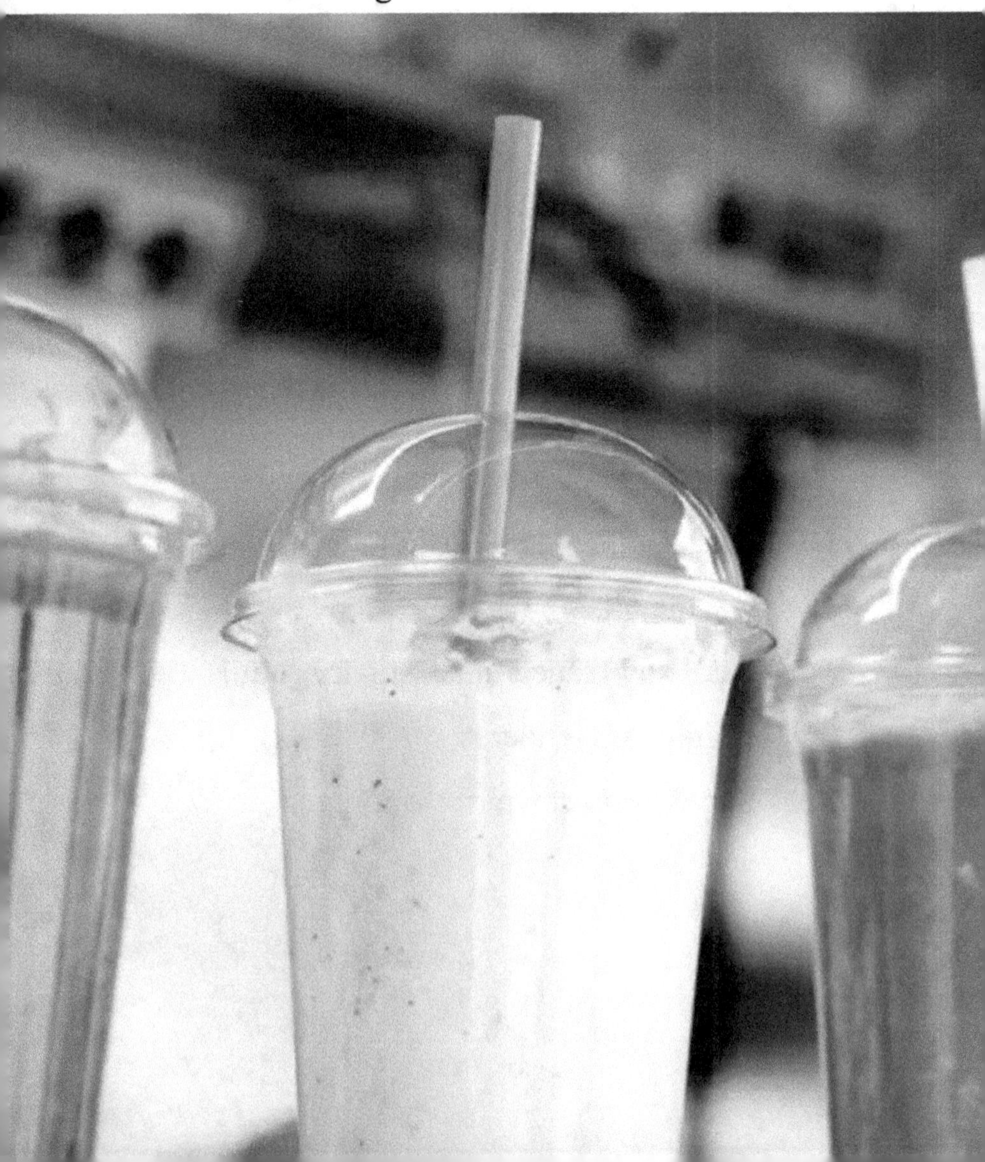

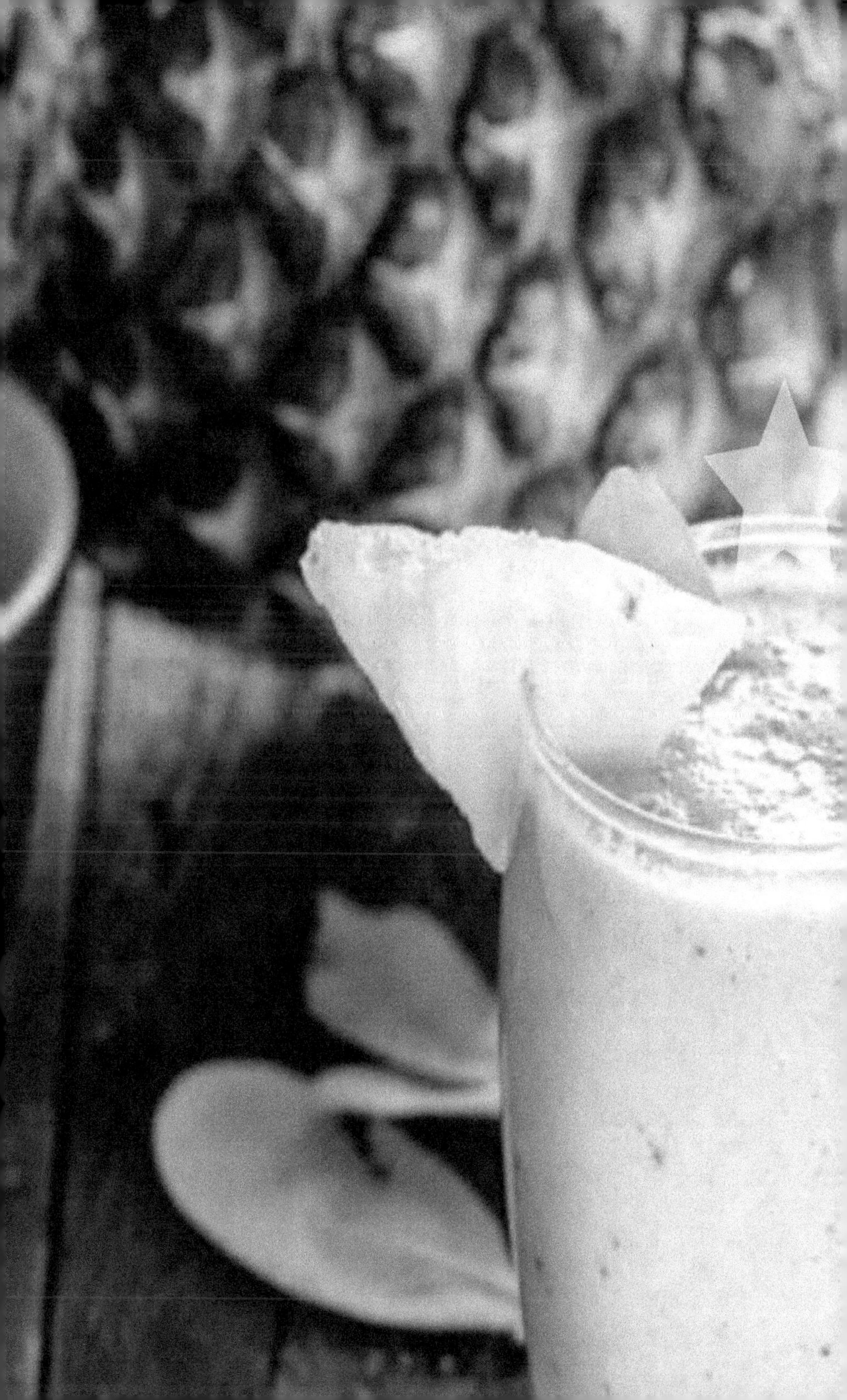

CONCLUSION

As we close the pages of this Anemia Diet Cookbook, we reflect on the journey we've embarked upon—a journey towards better health and vitality. This collection of recipes is more than just a guide to cooking; it's a beacon of hope for those affected by anemia, illuminating the path to a stronger, more energized self.

Through the incorporation of iron-rich foods, the enhancement of nutrient absorption, and the mindful selection of ingredients, we've learned that our diet can be a powerful ally in managing anemia. Each recipe has been crafted not only with flavor in mind but also with the intent to nourish and replenish the body.

Remember, the key to success in combating anemia lies in consistency and balance. It's about making informed choices, understanding the importance of each meal, and recognizing the role that food plays in our overall well-being.

As you continue to use this cookbook, let it serve as a reminder that every bite you take can be a step towards a healthier you. May these recipes bring color to your plate, strength to your body, and joy to your heart.